The
Child
Within

MARI HANES

The Child Within

*9 months of spiritual
preparation for the
woman in waiting*

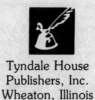

Tyndale House
Publishers, Inc.
Wheaton, Illinois

Library of Congress
Catalog Card Number 78-57967
ISBN 0-8423-0232-8, paper
Copyright © 1979
by Mari Hanes. All rights reserved.

Third Printing, May 1980
Printed in the
United States of America

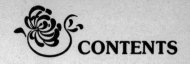
CONTENTS

7 Foreword

13 Conception

15 The First Month

25 The Second Month

35 The Third Month

45 The Fourth Month

53 The Fifth Month

61 The Sixth Month

71 The Seventh Month

81 The Eighth Month

89 Delivery

101 The Newborn

113 Bibliography

115 Personal notes

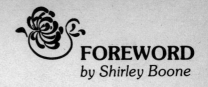

FOREWORD
by Shirley Boone

Over the past twenty years I've read many books dealing with bearing children and raising them. They offered all kinds of answers to physical and emotional needs. Recently there have been books on the market helping us with the spiritual demands of child-rearing and family life. Having gone through four pregnancies and having raised four daughters, I recognize that God's grace has seen me through many difficult situations, even though I've made mistakes. I'm so thankful for those who are digging into the Word and coming up with God's answers, so we can all avoid a lot of pitfalls.

Mari Hanes has filled a unique need by supplying spiritual answers for the pregnant woman. It's a positive approach to lift your spirits when you're feeling "heavy."

In a nation where many are obsessed with their right to abort an unborn child, it is refreshing to read words of wisdom from someone who wants to face the responsibility of "the child within."

The Child Within is timely, thought-provoking, and inspiring for the pregnant woman. I personally recommend it to all who are, or hope to be, expectant mothers.

There are days in your pregnancy
  when your heart fills with the warmth of joy
  and, like the flight of a pastel balloon,
    seems to float into heaven.

Your thrill at the thought of Life within
  is swallowed by the even greater
  anticipation
    of who that little life will be.

But there are other days—
  thankfully fewer—
  when physical and emotional pressures
    combine to rob you
  of your happiness and peace.

It is for those days that this study guide is
  written.

*Find comfort in knowing that your fears and
    worries are neither strange,
      nor unusual . . .
        Just as every healthy fetus develops
        according to a certain physical pattern,
      every expectant mother
        has in common with her sisters
          the need for many steps of inner growth.*

*As your baby develops physically within you,
    may you develop emotional and spiritual
      stability.*

      *Most of all,
          may you learn to draw on the enduring
          strength of a heavenly Father
        who promises
          to . . .*

        "Gently lead those that are with young."

          Isaiah 40:11

BEFORE YOU BEGIN:

More important than what is written in this book is what God will speak to your heart through his Word and prayer about your-own-and-special child within.

It is wisdom to keep a journal of your pregnancy.

Keep that journal and your Bible at hand as you begin this study guide.

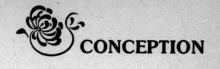 CONCEPTION

Great is our Lord, and of great
 power:
 his understanding is infinite.
The Lord is good to all:
 and his tender mercies are over
 all his works.
Let them praise the name of the
 Lord:
 for he commanded, and they
 were created.
        Psalm 147:5; 145:9; 148:5

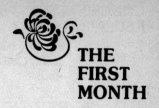

THE FIRST MONTH

The major development of the embryo takes place before a woman is even certain that she is pregnant:

A minute heart is pulsating and pumping blood. Backbone and spinal cord are forming. The digestive system is being created. Small buds appear, which will soon become arms and legs.

You saw me before I was born
*   and scheduled each day of my*
*   life*
*   before I began to breathe.*
Every day was recorded in your
*   Book!*
                    Psalm 139:16 (TLB)

CONCEIVING, RECEIVING

> *In every thing give thanks: for this is the will of God in Christ Jesus concerning you.*
>
> 1 Thessalonians 5:18

Babies are conceived under many different circumstances.

Some pregnancies are the result of months of planning and prayer which culminate in a conception that brings tremendous joy to both parents. Some pregnancies bring unexpected delight, and are as wonderfully surprising as an early Christmas would be to a four-year-old. Other pregnancies are not only unplanned, but unwanted, and for many valid reasons may fill the expectant mother's heart with dread and fear.

Whether your conception was by purpose or chance, there is one question which must be settled in these first weeks: *"Is the child within a part of God's will for my life?"*

There is a scriptural truth which will flood your heart with peace: your child was not conceived outside of the foreknowledge of your heavenly Father. God's words to your unborn infant are the same as his words to the prophet Jeremiah, "I knew you before you were formed within your mother's womb" (Jeremiah 1:5, TLB).

If you suspect that there is a child within, you can receive that tiny being as a part of God's will for your life. And his will, contrary to what many have thought, is a plan designed to bring about your *greatest happiness*. Have you had misgivings about God's blueprint for your life, secretly dreading what he may bring your way? If so, 1 John 4:18 will illuminate the reason:

> *We need have no fear of someone who loves us perfectly; his perfect love for us eliminates all dread of what he might do to us.* If we are afraid, *it is for fear of what he might do to us, and shows that* we are not fully convinced that he really loves us! (TLB).

Even if you are a woman who has been taught since childhood of a loving heavenly Father, you may not be fully convinced that he really loves *you, individually* and *unconditionally.* During pregnancy, perhaps more than at any other time of your life, you need to be *fully convinced* of his love. You need to rest in that love, allowing it to be the *stabilizing factor for your life,* and for the life of your family.

The message of God's love for the individual flashes like a neon light throughout the Bible, and we must *"believe him* when he tells us that he loves us dearly" (1 John 4:16, TLB). Understanding that God wants the best for you will enable you to believe the promise of his Word that, "All that happens to us is working for our good if we love God and are fitting into his plans" (Romans 8:28, TLB).

During pregnancy, changing hormones may place you on an emotional trampoline; at times you may not feel that God (or anyone else) really loves you. But remember, we base our faith on his love for us, not on our feelings, but on *fact* . . . the fact that his Word tells us so! In 2 Corinthians 5:7 we are told, "We walk by faith, not by sight." That means that our spiritual life is not based on our senses, which are inconsistent, but on God's Word, which is steadfast!

You can be certain that this pregnancy flowed from the hand of the One who loves you; One who also loves the child within. Your excitement over a baby may have been dimmed by your hesitation to bring him into a troubled world. From television, from news reports, from modern philosophers comes an easily absorbed fear of impending doom. Many women today are saying, "I'm afraid to have children because I'm concerned over what the future holds for them."

Christians are not immune to this fear. As believers, we understand that Christ's return to earth is imminent, and currently the study of "the last days" is extremely popular. Biblical prophecies, and the books dealing with them, are meant to urge unbelievers to prepare for the Second Coming. Yet recently these writings have had an adverse effect on some of God's children. Instead of waiting eagerly for the arrival of our Lord, and remembering that his Kingdom will bring indescribable peace and unending health, you may dread circumstances which may surround that event.

As a Christian, dread of the future should never be a reason for remaining childless! Scriptural principles are timeless, and the scriptural principle regarding Christians and conception is set forth in the 29th chapter of Jeremiah. As God's children faced exile in Babylon, the Holy Spirit spoke through the prophet and gave these instructions:

> Build homes and plan to stay; plant vineyards . . . Marry and have children, and then find mates for them and have

*many grandchildren. Multiply! Don't
dwindle away!* (v. 5, 6, TLB).

Then, in verse 11, God gave the concept of
his loving will which is reinforced by the New
Testament:

*For I know the plans I have for you, says
the Lord. They are plans for good and
not for evil, to give you a future and a
hope* (TLB).

In this portion of Scripture, God's children
are assured that:

A. He wants us to have families, and
B. He will bless and keep our families
no matter what world situation we
may face.

At this crucial time in your life, will you
allow the Holy Spirit to bring you to the point
of being *fully convinced* of his love for you
and for the child within? Will you embrace his
love with your heart, and not just with your
mind?

Before you begin the following study, go to
your Father in honest prayer. Hebrews 4:15,
16 urges you to approach him without fear.
Your relationship with him is dearly intimate;
you may call him, ". . . Abba, Father"
(Romans 8:15), and the best interpretation of
the Greek word *"abba"* would be "daddy" or
"papa"!

Ask the Lord to give you the confidence
that the fetus snuggled deep inside of you is a
part of his wonderful plan for your life. Next,
ask him to assure you that he also has a
wonderful plan for the child he is knitting
together. Then you will experience a surge of

thankfulness for the priceless gift of a child within.

> *Lo, children are an heritage of the Lord,*
> *and the fruit of the womb is his reward.*
> Psalm 127:3

FAITH BUILDERS

I can trust in God's love.

1. Study 1 John 4:9, 10. What is the greatest way in which God has said, "I love you"?

   <u>Sent His Son as a sacrifice</u>
   <u>for our sins</u>
   Have you received the gift of God's love by receiving his Son, Jesus Christ, as your personal Savior? <u>yes</u> ". . . if thou shalt confess with thy mouth the Lord Jesus, and shalt believe in thine heart that God hath raised him from the dead, thou shalt be saved" (Romans 10:9).

2. The Lord Jesus not only loves you: he understands you perfectly! How is he able to do this? (Read Hebrews 4:15.)

   <u>Because he has been tempted</u>
   <u>in every way.</u>

3. Sometimes, even after we become part of God's family, we feel like hiding from him because of sin. Your intimate relationship with your heavenly Father can be immediately restored. How? (Read 1 John 1:9.)

   <u>By confessing my sins</u>
   There is no need to ever feel far from God's love!

I can trust in God's will.

1. As a child of God, you are eager to discover his plan for your life, for you know that God's love flows out of God's wisdom. What does Isaiah 55:8, 9 teach us about the wisdom of God as compared to our plans and decisions?

   no comparison. He is so much greater + higher than me

   According to James 1:17, describe the quality of the things God wants to bring your way.

   good and perfect

2. Chapter 55 of Isaiah teaches the joy of living in the will of the Lord. Read verses 12, 13, and list some of the benefits and blessings.

   joy, peace, song, growth

3. If you are a mother-to-be in a lonely situation, single or separated from your husband, your pregnancy may have caused deep anxiety. Discover the Lord's special promise to you to become your Comforter, Counselor, and Protector. (Read Isaiah 54:4-8.) *Praise the Lord!*

I can trust in God's ways.

1. Think about the privilege of pregnancy. Name the source of your ability to conceive (Genesis 4:1).

   w/the help of the Lord

2. God's plan for man's earthly happiness

centers around what unit? (See Psalm
128: 3, 4.)

The Lord

3. Your ability to share in the kindling of a
    new being is an awesome gift from God,
    perhaps the way in which we are most "in
    his image." Write a statement expressing
    your trust in the will of God, and your
    thankfulness for the gift of this child.

*It is only by the grace
of God that I have
conceived. I trust the
Lord. He will bring it
to pass. Lord, thank you
for your gift of love, this
child.*

FURTHER DEVOTIONAL READING

The love of God. Deuteronomy 7:8; 9
Jeremiah 31:3; John 3:16; John 13:1;
John 15:13; John 16:27; Romans 5:8;
Romans 8:35; Ephesians 2:4, 5; 1 John 3:1

The blessing of children. Genesis 33:5; 48:9;
Joshua 24:3; Psalm 113:9; Psalm 127:3;
Psalm 127:4, 5; Psalm 128:3; Proverbs 17:6;
Isaiah 8:18

God's action during pregnancy. Job 10:8-12;
31:15; Psalm 119:73; 139:13-16;
~~Proverbs 26:10~~; Ecclesiastes 11:5;
Isaiah 42:5; 43:7; 44:2, 3, 21, 24;
45:11; 49:5; Zechariah 12:1;
Malachi 2:10; Acts 17:24-28;
Colossians 1:16, 17; Revelation 4:11

SUMMARY

The realization that your pregnancy can be used in God's wonderful and eternal plan for your life will bring you to the place of *thankfully accepting* the gift of your child within. As soon as you commit your life and the life of your baby to the Lord, he can "work all things together for your good!" You are now ready to develop emotionally as the fetus in your uterus develops physically.

Welcome to what can be the greatest experience of your life!

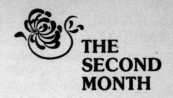

The embryo is now called a fetus and is $1^1/_8$ inches long, but weighs only $^1/_{30}$ ounce.

Limbs begin to show divisions into legs and feet, arms and hands, as bones are forming. The umbilical cord is distinctly visible. Internal organs are developing and functioning. Face and features begin to form: eyelids are fused.

As thou knowest not what is the way of the spirit,
    nor how the bones do grow
    in the womb of her that is
    with child:
even so thou knowest not the works of God
who maketh all.

                   Ecclesiastes 11:5

A
SPIRITUAL
EMBRYO

*Being confident of this very thing, that
he which hath begun a good work in
you will perform it until the day of Jesus
Christ.*

Philippians 1:6

At six weeks your pregnancy can be easily
confirmed by a visit to your doctor. You are
now certain that, in your excitement, you
have not just imagined the child within.

However your earthshaking announcement was made, the word is out. Snuggled
deep within the safety of your uterus, a tiny
person is now forming! Close friends hug their
congratulations, neighbors ask if you want a
boy or a girl, and your mother-in-law breathes
a contented, "Well, *finally!*"

Perhaps you feel like pinning a note to your
still-flat-and-inconspicuous tummy that says:
"An Announcement: There's a Baby in
Here!" You have officially joined the ranks of
the women-in-waiting. Your heart sings as
you go through your days, "In seven and a
half months I will be a mother! In seven and a
half months we will be three instead of two. In
seven and a half months . . ." Suddenly you
pause midsentence, for concern cascades
over your excitement. The nine months
gestation period which once sounded so long
is now clearly a very short time in which to
prepare yourself for parenthood.

There are a myriad details in physical
preparation for bringing an infant into your
home. But as a Christian believer, you
recognize that the reality of life is not only

physical, it is *spiritual.* Your heart cries out, "O God, as far as my spiritual and emotional development for being a mother is concerned, I am as incomplete as the embryo within me!"

This recognition of spiritual need is your only prerequisite for spiritual growth. Your realization of the need for God to develop your character, while his laws of nature are developing your baby, will set him free to do just that! The Word promises that he always hears the cry of a sincere heart.

Philippians 1:6 is a wonderful verse for every expectant mother. *The Living Bible* says it in this way: "God who began the good work within you will keep right on *helping you grow* in his grace until his task within you is finally finished . . ."

As soon as we commit our lives to God, he *does* begin a good work in us! Don't be impatient with yourself because you fail to reach spiritual maturity overnight. That would be as unnatural as having a baby that learned to walk and run in a few days! James 1:4 urges you to "let patience have her perfect work, that ye may be perfect and entire, wanting nothing." You must be patient with yourself, for your loving heavenly Father is patient with you. He is full of compassion, slow to anger, and of great mercy.

The crucial question is whether or not you are *spiritually hungry.* You shouldn't ask yourself, "Am I full-grown spiritually?" but rather, *"Am I growing?"* In 1 Peter 3:11 we are urged to "pursue a relationship with God" (Amplified).

To insure that growth, you will need a great deal of spiritual nourishment. During your pregnancy, your obstetrician will give you much advice regarding proper food, liquid intake, and your need of vitamins and minerals. The wise woman will decide to follow this advice implicitly. Recent studies have shown that not only the health, but also the intelligence of the child within depends upon your daily diet. The wise woman will also determine that her spirit, like the vulnerable fetus, is nourished continually. God has provided three nutrients for spiritual growth:

The milk of the Word
A newborn baby draws all of its needs from one substance: milk. Physicians have verified the fact that milk, especially a mother's milk, provides a perfectly balanced diet for the tiny infant. Scripture draws a parallel to this perfect diet:

> As newborn babes, desire the sincere milk of the word, that ye may grow thereby.

> 1 Peter 2:2

The Word of God provides a perfectly balanced diet for your spirit. "The whole Bible was given to us by inspiration from God and is useful to teach us what is true and to make us realize what is wrong in our lives. . . . It is God's way of making us well prepared at every point. . ." (2 Timothy 3:16, 17, TLB).

One of the saddest sights in the world is that of a grown woman who, because of accident or injury, has lost the use of her muscles to the point that she must relearn control in order to even feed herself. Equally sad, in God's eyes, is the sight of one of his daughters who does not know how to feed her spirit.

The strength of prayer
It does not matter if you are kneeling or washing dishes, if you whisper or speak loudly . . . are you talking to your Father each day? Throughout Scripture we are taught to call on him, for he is near! (See Isaiah 55:6.)

There is no need to face any of the concerns of pregnancy or the responsibilities of parenting alone. "Don't worry about anything; instead, *pray about everything;* tell God your needs and don't forget to thank him for his answers" (Philippians 4:6, TLB).

In prayer you have the privilege of talking to the all-powerful God who had the authority to speak the universe into existence. But you also have the privilege of talking to the *understanding Savior.* Remember the verses in Hebrews you studied last month?

> *This High Priest of ours understands our weaknesses, since he had the same temptations we do, though he never once gave way to them and sinned. So let us come boldly to the very throne of God and stay there to receive his mercy and to find grace to help us in our times of need.*

Hebrews 4:15, 16 (TLB)

Fellowship
"But if we are living in the light of God's presence, just as Christ does, then we have wonderful fellowship and joy with each other . . ." (1 John 1:7, TLB).

As a Christian, it is God's will for you to be part of a local church family. When the Word speaks of "fellowship," it means much more than sitting in a church service, or knowing other believers only on a "hello . . . good-bye" basis. Allow your Father to give you insight into a vital, living relationship with the Body of Christ. "All of you together are the one body of Christ and each one of you is a separate and necessary part of it" (1 Corinthians 12:27, TLB). If your life is lacking in true and deep fellowship, tell your Father your need. Ask him to add to your life dear friends who will give you the godly encouragement and support you need as a young wife and mother.

Perhaps the single most important step of preparation for delivery will be to find someone to act as a prayer partner, interceding with you throughout your labor.

"Can I grow to spiritual maturity?" you may have wondered. "Can I add to my personality the qualities of character that will make me a good mother?" The answer is yes—yes, as you follow God's plan of growth! He extends this promise to you as his daughter:

> Seek ye first the kingdom of
> God . . . *and all these things shall be*
> *added unto you.*
>
> Matthew 6:33

FAITH BUILDERS

The right attitude

1. King David was a man "after God's own heart." What was the attitude of David's heart which God found so pleasing? (See Psalm 42:1, 2.)

   <u>He "thirsted" for God</u>

2. The Apostle Paul also wrote of his

constant spiritual hunger. Put Philippians 3:13, 14 into your own words:

Leave the past and press on to the goal God has prepared for me, Jesus Christ.

3. Do you feel that your spiritual appetite needs to be stronger? Pause right now to ask God to do a special work in your heart. Remember: "For God is at work within you . . . helping you do what he wants" (Philippians 2:13, TLB).

The right action
Basically we are given two tools with which to build up our spirits:

1. We talk to God
   a. When do you have the privilege of praying?

      1 Chronicles 16:11 *Always*

      1 Thessalonians 5:17 *Continually*
   b. What is your attitude in prayer?

      2 Chronicles 7:14 *humility*

      Jeremiah 29:13 *hearts close to God*

      Psalm 95:2 *w/thanksgiving*
   c. What are we to do when we pray?

      Mark 11:24 *believe that what we ask for, we shall receive*

      James 1:6 *not doubt*
2. We let God talk to us
   a. How do we gain more faith?
      (See Romans 10:17.)

      listening to the word of Christ

b. What does the knowledge of God's
    Word bring about in our lives? (See
    2 Timothy 3:16, 17, TLB.)

teaching, rebuking, cor-
recting & training in
righteousness

c. The Bible deals with all aspects of
    life. Think about your own situation;
    list several areas of life about which
    you would like the Lord to speak to
    you as you study his Word.

_____

_____

_____

The right relationship
1. Just as your physical body provides
    nourishment for the fetus within you, a
    church body will provide nourishment for
    the embryo of your spiritual experience.
    Study Romans 12:5-8 and list the differ-
    ing ministries you will receive through
    consistent fellowship with other believers.

prophecy, serving, teaching,
encouragement, needs meeting
leadership, mercy

2. What will a good church family add to
    your life? (See Jeremiah 3:15.) *knowledge*
    & understanding
3. You are a busy woman in a busy society,
    and establishing a daily time of prayer
    and Bible study takes much discipline.
        Set up a time: God walked with Adam
    and Eve each evening; David called on
    God each morning; Paul and Silas were

good at praising God at midnight! What about you?

As you begin, set a realistic goal for yourself. (It is better to reach a small goal than to become so discouraged with a higher goal that you give up completely.) Perhaps at first your daily devotions will include only five minutes of prayer and a chapter from the Word. But whatever goal you set, *begin now!* The habit should be well established before you enter the hectic period of caring for a newborn infant.

FURTHER DEVOTIONAL READING

A woman of prayer. Psalm 55:17; Daniel 6:10; Matthew 6:6, 9; Matthew 26:41; Luke 11:9; Luke 18:1; Romans 8:26, 27; 1 Corinthians 14:15

A woman of the Word. Deuteronomy 8:3; Deuteronomy 11:18; Job 23:12; Psalm 119:11; Psalm 119:103; Jeremiah 15:16; Colossians 3:16; 2 Timothy 3:16; ~~1 Peter 1:21~~; 1 Peter 2:2

A woman of fellowship. Psalm 111:1; Psalm 119:63; Malachi 3:16; Matthew 18:20; Luke 24:15, 32; Acts 2:42; Philippians 1:3, 5; Hebrews 10:25; 1 John 1:7

SUMMARY

Deep inside your uterus is a tiny, but rapidly developing fetus. Within your body is another *treasure* which cannot be seen with the natural eye: your developing spirit. Both require nutritional care.

As the child within and your spirit are nourished, God's laws are set in motion. Growth is *natural* and *inevitable*. These months before delivery can add a quality to your life that will always remain with you. At the end of the gestation period, it is possible to be not only bulging with physical life, but brimming with spiritual life as well!

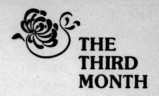

THE THIRD MONTH

The fetus is now 3 inches long and weighs about an ounce.

Hands and feet are fully formed; nails are distinctly present. External ears are evident. Eyelids are still fused. Tooth sockets and buds are forming in jawbones. Heartbeat can now be detected with special instruments.

Your baby may develop with head down, or continue to rotate until the last weeks of pregnancy. It lives its uterine life within the "bag of waters," which serves as an excellent shock absorber. The amniotic fluid in this sack is not stagnant; it is completely replaced eight times each day.

Happy shalt thou be, and it shall be well with thee.
He hath blessed thy children within thee.
                    Psalm 128:2b; 147:13b

> *For God hath not given us the spirit of fear; but of power, and of love, and of a sound mind. What time I am afraid, I will trust in thee.*
>
> 2 Timothy 1:7; Psalm 56:3

Before you were pregnant, you had no idea how the knowledge of your child within would consume you. Baby-to-be is your constant companion, not only in body, but also in thought.

Into your pleasant thoughts, like hostile aliens in a peaceful land, can come doubts and fears which turn daydreams into nightmares and rob you of the joy of pregnancy.

Obstetricians tell us that prenatal anxieties fall into three main categories: 1. Fear of the disfigurement or miscarriage of the fetus. 2. Fear of the pain involved in labor and delivery, and the possible loss of your attractiveness following the birth. 3. Fear regarding the future of the child (financial concern or anxiety over the world situation such as mentioned in chapter one). By far the most prevalent is the first category—the fear that something may go wrong with the child within.

At times you may wish you had skin so transparent that you could look in and get just a glimpse of how baby is doing. One frustrated woman even asked, "Why couldn't God have made human mothers like he made kangaroos, complete with a pouch on the outside where baby does most of its developing?"

The answer is that we could not resist attempting, however clumsily, to "help" the fetus along.

When we are afraid, we rush to "fix" the situation. *Fear breeds manipulators*. The way of the world is to manipulate, to contrive, to gain control in any way possible. But God's way is different.

He asks us to *trust*.

God is the only one who can knit together a new being. He couldn't allow us to get our hands on what must be his work, his alone. Your words to yourself must be the words of Psalm 62:5: "Wait thou only upon God."

Many fears about pregnancy, labor, and childbirth will be handled by obtaining *accurate information*. Instead of listening to the details of a neighbor's difficult delivery or to "old wives' tales," ask questions of your doctor, read available literature, and sign up *now* for a Prepared Childbirth class. (If you will not be accompanied in the labor room by your husband, Prepared Childbirth teachers will welcome a friend or your mother as your "coach.")

Momentary fear and concern is normal, for you are facing a totally new experience. But what if your fears turn into giants which torment you? *What is the source of tormenting fear?*

At the root of fear is usually a mental or emotional lie, for psychological studies show us that most fears have *no sound basis,* and focus on events which *never take place.* The Word of God tells us the source of these lies.

In 1 Peter 5:8 we see that, as God's children, we are the object of spiritual warfare waged by his enemy, the devil. In John, chapter eight, Jesus describes Satan as "the father of liars."

Your enemy endeavors to get you to accept lies and their resulting emotion—fear. Have you ever realized that the thoughts you "hear" in your mind can either be *accepted* (if they are according to God's promises) or *rejected?* Have you realized that some of the ideas planted in your mind are not your own? You do not have to accept tormenting giants of fear!

"Thou wilt keep him in perfect peace, *whose mind is stayed on thee:* because he trusteth in thee" (Isaiah 26:3). It is the peace of God which will free you from fear. It is the peace of God which will "keep your hearts and minds through Christ Jesus" (Philippians 4:7). In other words, the peace of God acts as a sentinel, standing guard at the gates of your mind. That peace can cushion your emotions and protect you just as surely as the amniotic fluid protects the child within!

You may have had an experience which placed concern in your mind, such as acquaintance with a woman who has miscarried. Yet miscarriage in the early months is an act of grace in itself, for experts tell us that it is almost always the result of an improperly developed fetus. If something is wrong, the Lord has set up the laws of pregnancy so that it is taken care of. If the problem lies in a woman's physical makeup, the Lord has promised to heal "the miscarrying womb." (See Genesis 49:25.)

It is a concrete reality that your baby is *safer now,* deep within the uterus, than it will ever be again! There have been cases of pregnant women who have been in auto accidents or have sustained bad falls, resulting in fractures of the limbs of their unborn babies. Yet those babies healed nicely in the womb without medical help, and were born perfectly healthy! God has placed the fetus in a controlled, bacteria-free environment.

Soon the infant will grow to a toddler who faces the threat of contagious diseases; then to a child who faces playground cuts and bruises; then to a teenager who faces the strain of dating years; then to a young adult who faces the challenge of independence. Sooner or later, you must learn to be a mother who places her trust in God. By his grace you can learn *now*.

Yes, God does ask you to do your part. In a few short weeks you will be holding your baby, feeding it, caring for it constantly. But now is not the time. If the child within were able to speak to you at this time he would whisper, "Mother, be at peace and let God knit me together. He truly knows what he is doing!"

FAITH BUILDERS

The source of fear
1. In John 8:32, Jesus promises us that we will find freedom by *knowing the truth*. One truth which is presented time and time again in the Scriptures is that God has an enemy, the devil. According to John 10:10, what three things does the devil endeavor to do?

   steal, kill & destroy

2. One of the things which the enemy would try to steal from you is your peace of mind. What method does he use for doing this? (As mentioned earlier, see John 8:44b.)

lying

3. Perhaps your mind has been filled with fearful thoughts such as:

> *Something is wrong with the child within.*
> *God doesn't care and will not answer my prayers.*
> *I will not be able to be a good mother.*

If so, recognize that at the root of these fears there are lies, and that at the source of these lies there is an enemy. What warning are we given in 2 Corinthians 2:11?

don't let Satan outwit or take advantage of you

4. Jesus came to mankind to show us God's love. In 1 John 3:8 we find another reason for his coming:

to destroy the devil's work

The source of serenity

1. We combat lies in the same way Jesus did when he confronted the devil in the wilderness. (See Luke 4.) We use *God's Word*. If you have been troubled by a

recurring fear, search the Scriptures and find a verse to dispel that particular fear:

_____

_____

_____

(Your Bible's concordance may be of help to you.)

2. Instead of allowing your mind to be filled with depressing fears, you can dwell on thoughts which will foster serenity. List the eight characteristics of the thought-life pattern which is shown in Philippians 4:8.

a. ~~truth~~ true

b. ~~nobility~~ noble (honest)

c. right (just)

d. pure

e. lovely

f. admirable (of good report)

g. excellent (virtue)

h. praiseworthy

3. What does 1 Timothy 4:7 say about "old wives' tales" and superstition?

have nothing to do with them

4. God provides his children with a suit of spiritual armor. Study Ephesians 6:14-17 to understand the components of your protective covering.

a. truth

b. _righteousness_

c. _peace_

d. _faith_

e. _salvation_

f. _sword of the Spirit, the word of God_

Choosing faith instead of fear
The Bible uses the example of a pregnant woman, Sarah, to define what faith really is!

> *What is faith? It is the confident assurance that something we want is going to happen. It is the certainty that what we hope for is waiting for us, even though we cannot see it. . . . Sarah, too, had faith, and because of this she was able to become a mother in spite of her old age, for she realized that God, who gave her his promise, would certainly do what he said.*
> Hebrews 11:1, 11 (TLB)

FURTHER DEVOTIONAL READING

God's will for healthy babies.
Deuteronomy 7:13-15;
Deuteronomy 28:1-11; Malachi 4:2

Women who set an example of faith and fearlessness. Sarah—Genesis 17:15;
Hebrews 11:1, 11; Esther—the book of Esther, esp. 4:16; Hannah—1 Samuel 1, 2

Your authority over God's enemy.
Zechariah 3:2; Luke 10:17, 19;

Luke 22:31, 32; John 12:30, 31;
Acts 5:16; 16:18; 19:12; Ephesians 4:27;
Ephesians 6:11, 12; 2 Thessalonians 2:8;
Hebrews 2:14; James 4:7; 1 John 3:8

Examples of needless fear. Matthew 14:30;
Matthew 17:6; Mark 4:38; Mark 5:33;
Mark 16:5; Luke 1:12

SUMMARY

You cannot yet see your child within. The
Lord cannot allow us to manipulate something as fragile as the fetus, so in his wisdom,
he seals the baby deep within the mother's
uterus. According to the verses we have
studied above, this is *exactly* the time to be a
woman of faith!

"Worry over nothing! Pray about everything!" (See Philippians 4:6.) Believe that
every tiny part of your baby-to-be is being
fashioned by a wise heavenly Father, for *in
faith there is freedom from fear.*

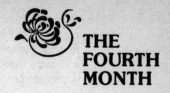

THE FOURTH MONTH

Your baby is now 6½ to 7 inches long and weighs 4 ounces.

Heartbeat is strong. Muscles are developed and active. Skin is bright pink and wrinkled. Eyes, ears, nose, and mouth approach typical appearance.

The uterus begins to enlarge noticeably with the developing fetus and can now be felt extending halfway up to the umbilicus.

You made all the delicate, inner parts of my body,
  and knit them together in my mother's womb.
Thank you for making me so wonderfully complex!
    It is amazing to think about.
Your workmanship is marvelous — and how well I know it.
          Psalm 139:13, 14 (TLB)

A STUDY
IN STABILITY

He shall feed his flock like a shepherd:
he shall gather the lambs with his arm,
and carry them in his bosom, and shall
gently lead those that are with young.

Isaiah 40:11

Through the miraculous process God has woven into his laws of nature, your body is undergoing tremendous change in order to nourish the child within.

Special hormones are being produced and your bloodstream is filled with an entirely new chemistry. The amount of some of the hormones in your system, such as crucially important estrogen, will more than *triple* before the baby is born. Your entire metabolism is readjusting; body fluid and blood volume increase, and your heartbeat will even quicken.

Perhaps you have read that these physical changes often bring emotional side effects. Friends have told you how touchy they were during pregnancy. "I burst into tears for the slightest reason," they confess, "my life was a string of emotional highs and lows for the entire nine months."

There are *five noticeable areas of change* with which you must cope simultaneously:
1. Cessation of menses   2. Breast and abdominal enlargement   3. Easy fatigability
4. Digestive problems such as heartburn, constipation, or nausea, and 5. Upheaval in the sexual drive. These changes *can* be tremendously upsetting, if you allow them to be, placing you on an emotional roller coaster and taking your husband and family along for the tearfully turbulent ride.

You may not always understand the things you are feeling. It is comforting to know that medical experts tell us that *all* women have both positive and negative attitudes toward pregnancy. Realize that the negative thoughts are not aimed at the baby, but rather *at your condition.*

You may go through stages of feeling depressingly unattractive. Combine a few flattering maternity outfits with interchangeable accessories; try a new hairstyle, weekly facials, and a daily shower. Most of all, remember to let your *inner radiance shine through.* The radiance which God has built into pregnancy will more than make up for your changing figure!

It's normal to spend much time thinking about yourself and the development of the baby. Yet be cautious that introversion doesn't cause you to withdraw from your husband or those around you. *Don't forget his needs in the preoccupation with your own needs.* Embrace your husband emotionally, just as you will soon embrace your infant. And as to your physical relationship, physicians agree that normal sexual intimacy can continue until the final six weeks of pregnancy. (See 1 Corinthians 7:5.)

The Word of God has much to say about each situation we may face in life—*even pregnancy.* Is getting up each day difficult for you because of morning sickness? "I shall be satisfied, when I wake, by beholding thy likeness." (See Psalm 17:15.) Do you feel drained of energy? "He giveth power to the faint; and to them that have no might he increaseth strength. . . . They that wait upon the Lord shall renew their strength" (Isaiah 40:29, 31). Do you have a need for God to touch you physically because of nagging back or leg aches? "I am the Lord who heals you. You can get anything—anything you ask for in prayer—if you believe" (Exodus 15:26b, Matthew 21:22, TLB).

Remember at all times during your pregnancy that *God understands you* and looks at you *tenderly.* When you feel emotionally shaky, never be ashamed to turn to him. "He is like a father to us, tender and sympathetic to those who reverence him. For he knows we are but dust" (Psalm 103:13, 14, TLB). He is our Good Shepherd, and Isaiah 40:11 tells us he ". . . shall *gently* lead those that are with young."

If you yearn for emotional stability, remember that your spirit and soul are so woven into your body that *emotional health and physical health cannot be separated.* Often emotional battles, even spiritual battles, are lost because physical resistance is low. In the first months of pregnancy you feel the need for extra rest. Don't fight fatigue! Climb into bed, or at least put your feet up and relax. "You chart the path ahead of me, and tell me where to stop and rest" (Psalm 139:3, TLB). This is an excellent time to open your Bible and receive the soothing ministry of God's Word.

Chapter five will deal further with the care of your body, for it is crucial that you be in top physical condition as you face childbirth and motherhood. The discipline of your physical being can only be accomplished as you learn to discipline your mind. *The disciplined mind produces emotional stability.*

Remember what you studied in chapter four about the source of tormenting fear? The thoughts of fear whispered to you by your spiritual enemy can either be accepted or rejected. So can other thoughts! Thoughts of self-pity. Thoughts of resentment. Thoughts of frustration or anger.

As you grew up, you settled into certain thought patterns. You may have never realized the importance of disciplining your mind, and as a result spend much time entertaining thoughts which harm your emotional stability. God warns us in Philippians 4:7, 8 that it is dangerous to let our minds wander aimlessly. This is why 1 Peter 1:13 tells us: "Gird up [get control of] . . . your mind."

There are two ways to live. We can live at the mercy of the situation in which we find ourselves or, as God's daughters, we can begin to *reign in life!*

> *All who will take God's gift of forgiveness and acquittal are kings of life [may reign in life] because of this one man, Jesus Christ.*
>
> Romans 5:17b (TLB)

Think of it! *A queen of life!* Not a roller-coaster rider. Not an emotional wreck. But a woman of *inner strength and stability* who can enjoy the precious season of her pregnancy.

FAITH BUILDERS

The reason behind the warning

1. According to Proverbs 23:7, what is the outward result of your inner thought life?

   _____

   _____

2. The thoughts which your spiritual enemy

would get you to accept fall into two main categories:

a. Your imagination is God-given, but *excessive daydreaming* can lead to discontent and restlessness. How does the Bible tell us to handle our thoughts? (See Jeremiah 4:14.)

wash evil from our hearts

What are we instructed to do in 2 Corinthians 10:5? *take captive every thought to make it obedient to Christ*

b. In Matthew 15:18-20, Jesus warns about *destructive thinking,* and lists several main categories of self-destructing thoughts. What are they?

_____

_____

Can you think of subtle thoughts which would fit in each of those major categories?

_____

Steps toward discipline

1. *Repentance* is always a prerogative for freedom from old habits. What action are we asked to take in 2 Corinthians 4:2?

renounce secret & shameful ways

2. What are we to do with a mind that wanders?

a. Ephesians 4:17 *no longer let it happen*

b. 2 Corinthians 10:5b *take out tho* *captive*

3. According to James 1:8, what is one of

the major causes of emotional instability?

doublemindedness

Are you facing a decision (about your faith, your future, etc.) which has not yet been resolved? Ask your Father to guide you in making this decision.

The positive provision

1. How can a woman who feels "shaky" in the area of emotional stability be transformed?

   a. Ephesians 4:22-24 *put off the old & put on the new*

   b. Romans 12:1, 2 *renew mind*

2. Through the power of the Holy Spirit, what can take the place of our undisciplined thought life? (See 1 Corinthians 2:16.)

   the mind of Christ

FURTHER DEVOTIONAL READING

Discipline of the mind. Job 42:2; Psalm 60:6; Psalm 139:2; Proverbs 4:23; Proverbs 21:2; Proverbs 22:11; Jeremiah 4:14; Ezekiel 11:5; Luke 6:45; Romans 12:3; Ephesians 4:17; Revelation 3:2;

Controlling my emotions. Proverbs 16:32; Acts 24:25; Romans 6:12; James 3:2; 2 Peter 1:5; Examples: Jeremiah 35:6; Daniel 1:8; 1 Corinthians 9:27

SUMMARY

Perhaps you have never before realized that the Lord wants you to be a *queen of life!* In 2 Corinthians 4:7 you are promised that through the resurrection power of Christ Jesus you can learn to reign!

The woman who can reign over her own thought life is the one who will be able to reign over her emotions. This month's priority: a disciplined mind!

> *In quietness and in confidence shall be your strength . . . And wisdom and knowledge shall be* the stability of thy times.
>
> Isaiah 30:15b; 33:6a

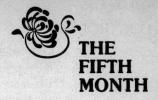

THE FIFTH MONTH

The baby is from 7 to 10 inches long and weighs from 8 to 9 ounces.

Internal organs are maturing at astonishing speed. A covering like peach fuzz appears over the entire body. At the end of the month, hair begins to grow on the baby's scalp.

But the very hairs of your head are all numbered.
Thus saith the Lord, thy Redeemer, and he that formed thee from the womb, I am the Lord that maketh all things.
        Matthew 10:30; Isaiah 44:24

IN CONTROL

> *A [person] without self-control is as*
> *defenseless as a city with broken-down*
> *walls.*
>
> Proverbs 25:28

Your responsibility toward your developing fetus is to provide it with a healthy environment. To do this, you must maintain constant vigilance toward your own health.

Like most women, you probably left the obstetrician's office following your first pregnancy exam armed with booklets on good nutrition, a prescription for prenatal vitamins, and the strong determination to get proper foods, plenty of rest, and daily exercise. At first it sounded like fun! Yet now that several months have elapsed, steak and salad may have given way to pizza and cokes, the "daily" vitamins may be remembered only once a week, and when it comes to exercise, you probably tell yourself, "I'll take a long walk tomorrow . . ."

How would you rate yourself in the area of self-control?

Are you well disciplined? Are you disgustingly undisciplined? Or, like most of us, are you out of control, then in control, and then disappointingly out again?

In Proverbs 25:28, a person lacking self-discipline is compared to an Old Testament city without the security of strong outer walls. In those times the doom of an unprotected city was certain. In other words, a woman who is out of control is the target of attack: in mind, in soul, and in body. In chapter 4 we talked about being a queen in life. Let's see what the Word has to say about reigning over our bodies.

There came a time in the history of Israel when Jerusalem was conquered by the Babylonians and the mighty walls of that city were broken down. Under the leadership of the prophet Nehemiah, 142 years later, the Jews were returning to their capital. What was the first thing they did? "Come, let us *build up the wall* of Jerusalem, that we be no more a reproach" (Nehemiah 2:17). The Israelites knew that without the walls to protect them, they would be at the mercy of surrounding hostile tribes.

Jerusalem is the city of which God said, "Sing praises to the Lord, which dwelleth in Zion" (Psalm 9:11a). After the coming of Christ, through the power of the Holy Spirit, God promises to actually dwell in the hearts of his children. "I will dwell in them, and walk in them; and I will be their God, and they shall be my people" (2 Corinthians 6:16b). As a dwelling place of the Lord, Jerusalem can actually be a picture, a symbolic example, of the life of a Christian. Just as it was the will of God for Zion to be protected by fortified walls, God wants to erect walls of self-control in your life.

You may feel that your "walls" are a hopeless rubble. Perhaps you have been lacking in discipline all of your life, and this lack has only been magnified by your condition. (There is a unique craving for foods which occurs in pregnancy; this is known as pica.) You may have struggled with a weight problem, or with facing your housework and necessary chores, or with the myriad of responsibilities that come your way. You may be thinking, "Certain areas of my life have gotten away from me and I want to get them in control—but my motivational powers are *zilch!*" Like the Apostle Paul, you cry, "I don't understand myself at all, for I really want to do what is right, but I can't" (Romans 7:15, TLB).

There *is* an answer! Paul found it—*you* can find it! He asked, "Who will free me from my slavery . . .?" Then he recorded the answer: "Thank God! It has been done by Jesus Christ our Lord" (Romans 7:24, 25, TLB).

You see, Jesus did not just tell us how to live and then give us a farewell pat-on-the-back and say, "Lots of luck!" He didn't leave us to struggle along on our own . . . he promised an unlimited, ever-available power source.

The Holy Spirit.

Through the miraculous indwelling of the Holy Spirit, your pregnancy, and your entire life, can become a fortified city. Building on the foundation of the Rock of Jesus Christ, the Spirit will patiently rebuild your willpower. Allow him to add divine force to the strength of your own determination, for when an area of our physical desire is out of control, Philippians 3:19 says that it actually becomes a *god* which we worship.

Satan wants you to be out of control, and therefore at his mercy. God wants you to be *in control,* and therefore able to:

maintain your proper weight,
care for your body and the developing
child within through rest and exercise,
accomplish all of those things which a
woman in waiting needs to accomplish.

Last month you began to discipline your mind according to God's Word. Now you are ready for steps of outward discipline. Just as

Romans 8:5, 6 applies to ruling as a queen over your mind, you can also exercise *bodily control* like a reigning spiritual queen of life!

Biblical perspective

1. According to Proverbs 16:32, what is the value placed on self-control?

   better than taking over a city

2. The Bible uses the word "discipline" when speaking of self-control, and teaches that discipline determines what kind of woman you become. (See Proverbs 4:23.) What are two of the results of self-control?

   Proverbs 12:24 *rule*

   Proverbs 10:4; 21:5 *profit & wealth*

3. Proverbs 23:21, 22 warns against what area of undiscipline which specifically applies to the woman in waiting?

   eating too much garbage

4. In Isaiah 37:3, what is the major concern as you look toward delivery? *strength*

A biblical picture

1. The rebuilding of the walls surrounding Jerusalem serves as an illustration of rebuilding areas of our lives. According to Zechariah 4:7, how was Nehemiah to accomplish this monumental task? _____

   God's blessing

2. Zechariah 4:7 is understood as we have a clear definition of the word "grace." Grace means "the working of God

through his mercy." According to 2 Corinthians 12:9, what areas of our life provide perfect opportunities for the working of God's power?

our weaknesses

3. How is God's power made available to help us control the desires of our bodies? (See Romans 8:13.)

through the Holy Spirit

Personal application

1. Read about the special fruit of the Spirit that is listed in Galatians 5:22, 23. One of the fruits is temperance, meaning "balanced, self-controlled living." In what area of your life do you need the Spirit to bring about balance?

exercise

2. As in all areas of spiritual growth, self-control will develop on a continual, not an instantaneous, basis. What does 1 Corinthians 9:25 speak to your heart?

I need to be in constant "training"

3. As mentioned in this chapter, when an area of our life is out of control, it becomes a "god" to us. Discover the promise in Isaiah 26:13 about the personal freedom the Spirit can bring to your life.

FURTHER DEVOTIONAL READING

God's will concerning my diet. Psalm 141:4; Proverbs 23:1, 2, 20; Proverbs 25:16, 27;

Isaiah 55:2; Luke 10:8; Luke 12:22;
Luke 21:34; 1 Corinthians 10:25;
1 Corinthians 10:31; 1 Timothy 4:4

Physical rest. Isaiah 11:10; Isaiah 28:12;
Jeremiah 30:17; Zephaniah 3:17;
Matthew 11:28

In control. Matthew 5:29; Romans 6:6;
Romans 13:13; Romans 14:21;
1 Corinthians 9:25, 27; Galatians 5:16;
Colossians 3:5; Titus 2:2; 1 Peter 2:11;
1 Peter 3:10; 1 Peter 4:2

The power source. Ezekiel 36:27;
Matthew 3:11; Luke 11:13; John 15:5;
Acts 1:8; Acts 2:38; Romans 8:11;
1 Corinthians 3:16

SUMMARY

It is a fact of medical science that people are
susceptible to certain illnesses when their
resistance is low. *Self-discipline* is the resisting
wall between your health and the physical
problems that can result from lack of ade-
quate exercise, rest, and nutrition. It is also
the protecting wall between you and the mental and emotional assaults mentioned in
previous chapters.

How will we be able to discipline our children if we have not learned to discipline
ourselves? This month's priority: Control over
my body! With God's help, I am able!

> But we have this treasure in earthen
> vessels, that the excellency of the power
> may be of God, and not of us.
> 2 Corinthians 4:7

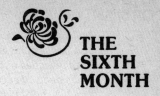

THE
SIXTH
MONTH

Your baby has now grown to be 10 to 13 inches in length.

The muscles are more active, and because of the baby's size, you often feel movement! Nails form on the tiny fingers and toes. At the end of the month, eyelids are separated.

Thou art worthy, O Lord, to receive glory and honour and power: for thou hast created all things, and for thy pleasure they are and were created.
Revelation 4:11

THE GIFT
OF SIGHT

*We know about these things because
God has sent his Spirit to tell us, and his
Spirit searches out and shows us all of
God's deepest secrets. But the spiritual
man has insight into everything.*
1 Corinthians 2:10, 15 (TLB)

The womb is neither dark, nor silent.

During this sixth month, the child within's previously fused eyelids are finally separated. Although the uterus is lacking in bright light, the baby's eyes *do* begin to open and shut, and he is able to see!

At the same time, your baby is acquiring a sense of hearing. The sounds he hears range from the rhythm of your heartbeat and the sound of your voice to the crash and vibration of outside street noises.

How rapidly the fetus has developed from a basic embryonic stage to this point of amazing ability! Just as your unborn infant is acquiring perceptive ability, you need to be acquiring spiritual perception, spiritual insight.

Many women do not realize that the spiritual dimension is every bit as real as the physical dimension of life. In fact, the spiritual dimension is *more real:* it existed before the physical world and will remain after this world has ended. Many rely solely on their natural abilities, such as sight and hearing. As a woman who has a relationship with the living God, and who is receiving spiritual nourishment as studied in chapter 2, you can operate with the advantage of an added dimension.

We live in a time when many of our concepts of how life should be lived are pressed on us by a society which operates outside of the principles of God. The Bible refers to the unbeliever as the "natural man" and says:

> *The man who isn't a Christian can't understand and can't accept these thoughts from God, which the Holy Spirit teaches us.*
> 1 Corinthians 2:14 (TLB)

This is why Romans 12:2 warns us:

> *Don't let the world around you squeeze you into its own mould, but let God remould your minds from within, so that you may prove in practice that the plan of God for you is good (Phillips version).*

This sixth month of pregnancy is one of great excitement, for sometime between the fifth and sixth months you have experienced "quickening." Your child within has moved all along, but now he has grown to the point that you can feel *life!* In the same way, as spiritual insight grows, there are things of power in the spiritual dimension which God can "quicken" in your understanding. Scriptural concepts which have seemed to be only tradition or mere words can leap to life!

What are some of these principles which are especially meaningful to the woman in waiting?

Positive confession: In the fourth month of pregnancy, you studied verses from God's Word about emotional stability. Your spiritual exercise was to discipline your mind . . . rejecting tormenting fear or worry or other emotions which are not God-inspired. You discovered the principle of filling your mind with "Whatsoever things are good. . . ." Now it is time to take another step of spiritual maturity: *speaking by faith.*

This is one area in which spiritual insight will show you a way that greatly differs from the way of the world. The world would cast you into the mold of a woman who speaks negatively. Have you found yourself making statements such as, "I'll probably be just like my mom and have an unusually long labor"? With the psalmist, the woman in waiting needs to pray, "Set a watch, O Lord, before my mouth." (141:3).

Jesus said that by our *words* we will be justified, or by our words we will be condemned. (See Matthew 12:37.) In Mark 11:23, he dealt further with the principle of positive confession: *"Ye shall have what ye say."*

In the fifth chapter of 1 Timothy, verse 13, Paul warned that one quality of foolish women is that they speak ". . . things which they ought not." Be a wise woman, with the spiritual insight to speak with *faith* about the birth of your baby. . . .

> *I'm looking forward to the birth of the child within.*
> *I know God promises to be with me continually, and so I am not afraid.*
> *I know God will bless me with calmness and strength.*

This is *not* just positive thinking. It is the scriptural principle of verbally claiming God's promises. Remember, "The word [of faith] is nigh thee, even in thy mouth. . ." (Romans 10:8).

The power of praise: Open your spiritual ears to hear what the Holy Spirit wants to teach you about the exercise of praise.

Is praise a word that you associate only with the Thanksgiving holiday or Handel's Hallelujah Chorus? If the idea of praise seems foreign to you, if your only involvement in praise has been as a part of formal church liturgy, the Bible can open your eyes to an entirely new concept.

To praise God means to speak or sing of your thankfulness. It can flow from your heart during your devotional time, as you do your housework . . . any time! This exercise is similar to physical exercise; you may not feel like it until you actually begin. But with practice, praise will become a well-developed spiritual response.

1. Praise God for *who he is.* "O Lord, you are worthy to receive the glory and the honor and the power" (Revelation 4:11, TLB). This lifts you out of the trap of too much introspection; physicians tell us that our bodies operate more smoothly if we don't concentrate on every minute twinge.

2. Praise God for *what he has done.* "You have created all things. They were created and called into being by your act of will" (Revelation 4:11b). Thank him for the conception of your child. Thank him for your spiritual growth in the past weeks.

3. Praise God for *what he will do.* Hannah and Elisabeth, along with other women of faith whose stories are recorded in the Bible, thanked God for their children *before* they were born.

Psalm 22:3 teaches us that God inhabits the praises of his people! The woman who learns to praise experiences a special awareness of his presence.

Communion: Many of us have received the Lord's Supper regularly since childhood. This month, allow your Father to open your eyes to a new understanding of communion, for this powerful symbol of Christ's resurrection is especially meaningful to the woman in waiting and the child within.

> *For every time you eat this bread and drink this cup, you are* representing *and* signifying *and* proclaiming the fact of the Lord's death [and resurrection] until he comes [again].
>   1 Corinthians 11:26 (Amplified)

The true meaning of communion is the proclamation of the resurrection power! When received with understanding, it can be a dynamic instrument of physical and emotional health for the believer. Verse 30 of 1 Corinthians 11 even goes so far as to tell us that some early Christians suffered weakness and illness because they didn't perceive the tremendous significance of communion.

Think of this truth as it applies to your baby. You are already well aware that everything which enters your system travels through the placenta and into the system of the child. This is why a balanced diet is so crucial, and why you must be cautious of even the mildest medication. When you receive the bread and juice of communion, some of the digested molecules *literally* become a part of the baby, proclaiming the fact of the Lord's resurrection power, the fact of his wholeness, to the body of the little one!

For the woman who bears a new life within her, the celebration of communion becomes much more than ceremony or tradition.

THE GIFT OF DISCERNMENT

In the Bible, the ability to see and hear in the spirit is called *discernment.* Discernment is the quality which enables us to see things as God sees them.

God-given discernment will enable you to see a situation as it really is—to deal with the *root* of a problem instead of only its symptoms.

An example of this is the story of Celia, a lovely young woman who said, "I don't want my husband to go through delivery with me because Don is the nervous type, and I'm sure he wouldn't make it." One day during devotions, the Holy Spirit whispered to her heart that the real fear was that she might take the stress of labor out on her husband, snapping at him and perhaps ruining the joy of their teamwork. As the couple discussed her fear, she was reassured by her husband of his understanding love. They held hands and prayed about it. When the time of her delivery arrived, Celia and Don worked together as a perfect unit during the birth of their baby girl.

Godly wisdom, godly discernment, will keep the world around you from "pressing you into its mold." As motherhood approaches, let the Lord be the one who dictates your lifestyle. See things *his way,* not man's way, in such areas as how to build your marriage and how to discipline your children.

Jesus named the Holy Spirit as "The Teacher." "But I will send you the Comforter—the Holy Spirit, the source of all truth. He will come to you from the Father and will tell you all about me" (John 15:26, TLB). The Spirit hears us as we ask him. . .

> *Open my eyes to see wonderful things in your Word.*
>
> Psalm 119:18 (TLB)

FAITH BUILDERS

God-given insight

1. How does 1 Corinthians 1:25 compare our natural wisdom with the wisdom of God? God's foolishness is wiser then man's wisdom

2. What does the Word give as (a) the characteristics of God-given wisdom, and (b) the simple formula for obtaining that wisdom?

   a. _____

   _____

   b. fearing God

3. What will be the result of your receptive (teachable) attitude?

   to be wise

Spiritual "quickening"

1. Study Mark 11:23, 24, then write a statement of *positive confession* regarding the child within.

   _____

2. *Praise* is a powerful spiritual principle.

What concept from Psalm 100:4 can you add to your daily prayer times?

Thanksgiving & praise

We learn to praise not only by feeling, but by faith—see Psalm 107:22.

3. According to Matthew 26:26, 28, what do the two elements of the *communion* service represent?

Christ's blood & body

What powerful message is proclaimed by this two-fold ceremony?

1 John 1:7 _blood purifies us from every sin_

Isaiah 53:5 _healing_

Personal application

1. Modern psychology extols the benefits of self-analysis. Why is God's gift of discernment (insight) more beneficial? (See Hebrews 4:12, 13.)

nothing is hidden from God's sight

2. Do you have a problem or question you have been unable to get to the root of? Ask God for the insight to look past the surface issue and understand the real need.

_____

_____

FURTHER DEVOTIONAL READING

Praise. Deuteronomy 8:10;
1 Chronicles 16:25; Psalm 9:11; Psalm 33:2;

Psalm 35:28; Psalm 67:3; Psalm 113:3;
Isaiah 42:12; Acts 2:47; Colossians 3:15;
1 Thessalonians 5:18; Hebrews 13:15;
1 Peter 2:9

Speaking by faith (positive confession).
Mark 11:23, 24; John 16:23, 24;
1 John 3:21, 22; 1 John 5:14, 15

God-given insight and discernment.
Proverbs 3:19; Ecclesiastes 7:19; 2:26;
Isaiah 11:2; Daniel 2:20, 21; Matthew 13:54;
Luke 2:40; 21:15; Romans 11:33;
1 Corinthians 1:25; Colossians 2:3;
2 Timothy 3:15; James 1:5; Examples:
1 Kings 4:31; 10:3

SUMMARY

In contrast to the early months of pregnancy,
now your baby makes you continually aware
of his presence. The fetus has gained weight
and increased in size so that you now have
the pleasure of feeling the stir of life within.

At the same time, are you allowing God to
add weight to your spiritual life? Are you
understanding the power in scriptural principles such as positive confession, praise, and
communion?

Every woman is concerned about looking
attractive during her pregnancy, and today
can enjoy the blessing of flattering maternity
outfits. Don't forget about the lovely clothing
that is available for your spirit!

> *Beauty for ashes,*
> *the oil of joy for mourning,*
> *the garment of praise*
> *for the spirit of heaviness.*

Isaiah 61:3

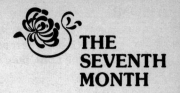

THE SEVENTH MONTH

The weight of your child within
has doubled since last month.

Skin is wrinkled and red, but
fatty tissue begins to form beneath
it. During this last trimester, the
fetus receives immunity to many
germs he will encounter as a
newborn.

*But now, O Lord, thou art our
Father:
we are the clay, and thou our
potter;
and we all are the work of thy
hand.*

Isaiah 64:8

PREPARING
A HOME

> *We should make plans — counting on*
> *God to direct us. Commit your work to*
> *the Lord, then it will succeed.*
>
> Proverbs 16:9, 3 (TLB)

When God created man in his image, he gave
us the gift of a free will and tremendous
creative potential. At no time in life are
creative decisions more *fun* than when you
are preparing your home for a new baby!
Though you may not fit into the category of a
traditional "bootie-knitter," in as many ways
as possible you are busily building a nest for
your child within.

God wants to be your Partner in the
preparation! His Holy Spirit can work
alongside you, assisting you with wise advice.
While you are working through the following
list of things-to-do-and-decisions-to-make,
get to know the Lord as your Counselor! "His
name shall be called Wonderful, *Counselor,*
The mighty God, The everlasting Father, The
Prince of Peace" (Isaiah 9:6b).

A. *"Prepared Childbirth" training:* Both you
and your husband will profit from attending
some type of childbirth training course, which
is usually begun in this seventh month.
Whether your delivery is completely natural
or aided by anesthesia, fear will dissolve as
you understand the entire birth process.
Labor will be much easier with the help of
relaxing exercises and breathing techniques.
According to Proverbs 27:12, the wise
woman is the one who is well prepared for
what lies ahead.

The classes will also enable your husband

to remain with you in the delivery room, strengthening you and sharing the indescribably poignant moment of the birth of your child. "Two are better than one . . . and a threefold cord is not quickly broken" (Ecclesiastes 4:9, 12). Your husband and your Lord will be the constant companions who unite with you to bring forth your child.

B. Child care preparation. If your experience with infants is lacking, your concern over delivery may be dwarfed by your concern over how to care for the baby when you bring him home. Don't panic! Use the next few weeks to give yourself a crash course on the care of infants. Many community groups, such as the Red Cross, offer brief, yet excellent classes. Now is also the time to purchase a reliable child care book (Be sneaky: look up steps A, B, and C for those questions you feel too embarrassed to ask anyone, such as "What *does* one do with soiled diapers?").

Best of all, expose yourself to the real thing! Visit friends with babies or volunteer for a few turns in the church nursery or day-care center. "Get all the [godly] advice you can and be wise the rest of your life" (Proverbs 19:20, TLB).

C. The nursery and layette. Your head will swim as you look over the list of suggested baby furniture and clothing. Where do you begin? What guidelines does the Word of God offer for this part of your preparation?

You'll love assembling a soft, tiny wardrobe, choosing baby furniture, and working with your husband to repaint that fantastic "find" you made at a garage sale (with lead-free paint, of course!). Enjoy every moment!

But don't go overboard—baby will quickly outgrow the wee shirts and gowns; and *convenient* and *durable,* instead of super-deluxe, should be the standard for nursery equipment.

Your devotional reading for this month includes Proverbs' description of the Model Wife and Mother. A major trait of her character is *practical* wisdom:

> *She looks after the needs of her household, and is never idle* (31:27).
> *She considers each purchase before buying it* (31:16).
> *She is energetic, a hard worker and "watches for bargains"* (31:18, TLB).

Practical wisdom is the natural outworking of true spiritual wisdom! The Lord literally wants to "teach you to profit." (See Isaiah 48:17.)

"Remember, your Father knows exactly what you [and your child within!] need even before you ask him" (Matthew 6:8, TLB). Jesus said:

> *[Don't] be of anxious [troubled] mind— unsettled, excited, worried and in suspense . . . your Father knows that you need them. Only aim at . . . and seek after His kingdom, and all these things shall be supplied to you also.*
> Luke 12:29-31 (Amplified)

D. Acquaint yourself with hospital procedures. Now is the time to find answers to any questions you have about what to do when the Big Moment arrives. The hospital where you plan to deliver will gladly welcome you and your husband on a tour of the maternity ward. Find out about billing procedures so that financial red tape will not detract from the enjoyment of your newborn; claim the promise that "God will supply all your needs according to His riches in glory!" (See Philippians 4:19.)

If you wish to have "rooming in" privileges, make arrangements in advance. Check on *when* and *how* your physician wishes to be notified when labor begins. Along with his phone number and those of close relatives, be ready to call the special Christian friends who have agreed to support you in prayer throughout the birth.

If you are planning to deliver in your own home, it is *especially important* to have everything ready with ample time to spare. The majority of babies are born within three days of the estimated due date—but there's always the chance your child within will come early.

Have you arranged to have help during the first days with your tiny infant? Whether you choose a relative or a neighbor, this blessed person may not do everything the way you would; but receive her help gladly. It is a scriptural principle for the older women to teach the younger women.

E. Nursing or formula. Today more and more physicians recommend breast feeding; it is more *economical,* as well as the easiest way to feed your infant. The Lord has marvelously equipped you to provide baby with a diet which is precisely balanced nutritionally, more easily digestible, and provides a definite immunity to childhood diseases. In Bible times, children were often nursed for several years. Isaiah 66:11 compares a time of peace in Israel with the tremendous comfort a baby receives from nursing at his mother's breast.

You may run into a few complications, the most common being a slow-up in milk supply or in the "let-down reflex" due to emotional or physical stress. In previous chapters you have already encountered the remedy for an emotional crisis: take it straight to Jesus!

Add to your baby book the purchase of a guide for breast feeding (Karen Pryor's *Nursing Your Baby* is excellent—or your obstetrician may offer a free handbook). It's best to be well read *before* you hold that hungry little person in your arms! And if you begin to toughen your nipples now, you'll be ready to nurse your child.

Unfortunately, breast feeding is not only "in" at this time . . . for some women it is becoming a cult with religious fervor. If, for some reason, you decide to use formula, there is *no need to feel condemned.* Remember, the *love* and *cherishing* you give your baby is far more important in God's eyes than the source of his milk!

More crucial than the physical environment which surrounds your children is the emotional environment of your home. A stable, secure home life flows from a stable, secure marriage. The best way to prepare your nest is to strengthen that love relationship.

Don't try to place on a child the heavy responsibility of "bringing you closer." If there have been problems in communication, if there are hurts or misunderstandings to be dealt with, deal with them *before* baby arrives. Pray for strength, as children will place greater demands on your union. Perhaps you need to consider seeking help from your pastor or other experienced counselors. If you seek counsel, remember the Word's instruction to "seek the advice of *godly* men."

Even the best of marriages will profit from some of the excellent readily available books on the Christ-centered marriage. Determine to *grow* in the relationship with the man God has given you even as you have determined to grow in your relationship with him! Love in marriage can be continually refreshed, for love springs from God.

With zest and enthusiasm, face the creative challenge of preparing the nest. *"Commit your work to the Lord, then it will succeed"* Proverbs 16:3, TLB).

FAITH BUILDERS

The scriptural principles.

1. What will insure the stability of the home you are preparing for your baby? (See Matthew 7:25; 1 Corinthians 3:11.)

    <u>having our foundation built on Jesus Christ</u>

2. Your marriage relationship will be strengthened as you follow God's scriptural instructions.

    a. What challenge to wives is given in Ephesians 5:22-24 and Titus 2:4, 5?

        <u>submit to and love your husband</u>

    b. Submission is for your protection, not for your degradation. What is the even more sobering challenge given

77

to husbands? (See Ephesians 5:25, 28; 1 Peter 3:7.)

love their wives as Christ loves the church

Personal application.

1. Chapter 31 of Proverbs describes a woman who is praised by both children and husband. (See verse 28.) Translate into modern terms the practical activities through which she ministers to her family.

   trust, meet husbands needs

   a. *help him, not hinder him*
   b. *makes clothes, shops, prepares meals, gardens, watches for bargains, decorates*
   c. *house, she makes things to sell, she is wise, watches*
   d. *over household*
   e. *not lazy, gives instruction*

2. According to Proverbs 21:9 and 25:24, what is the most destructive trait that can be found in a wife?

   being quarrelsome

   In a parent? (See 1 Samuel 3:13.)

   failed to discipline children

3. What effect can your life have on the faith of your family? (See 1 Peter 3:1, 2.)

   win them to Christ

4. In what way can you strengthen your marriage?

   _____

   Make this a matter of continuing prayer throughout the month.

Practical preparation.

1. There are two improper extremes to be avoided in the preparation of your nest.

    a. Proverbs 18:9; 6:6-8 *laziness*
    (God can supply motivation—see
    1 Thessalonians 4:1.)
    b. Matthew 6:19; 1 Timothy 6:10

    ___↑___↑___↑_____

    (Extravagance and overspending can
    point to insecurity—see Hebrews
    13:5.)

2. Do you feel lacking in creative ability? Are you concerned that you don't know how to do many things? (Sewing, decorating, etc.) Study Exodus 31:3, 4! _____

    _____

3. What is one way the Lord will provide your baby with material blessings? (See Isaiah 48:17.)

    God will teach us what is best.

FURTHER DEVOTIONAL READING

The book of practical wisdom—Proverbs.
(There is a chapter for each day of this month!)

God provides for our needs. Job 38:41;
Psalm 1:3; Psalm 23:5; Psalm 31:19;
Psalm 78:20; Proverbs 6:8; Isaiah 30:23;
Amos 9:13; Malachi 3:10; Matthew 14:20;

Ephesians 3:20; Examples: 1 Kings 17:6, 16;
2 Kings 4:6; Philippians 4:19

The solid home. Genesis 2:24;
Genesis 29:20; Deuteronomy 4:9;
Proverbs 18:22; Song of Solomon 8:7;
Colossians 3:19; 1 Timothy 3:4;
1 Timothy 5:4; Titus 2:5; Hebrews 13:4

SUMMARY

"Every wise woman buildeth her house. . . .
Through wisdom is an house builded; and by
understanding it is established. And by
knowledge shall the chambers be filled with all
precious and pleasant riches" (Proverbs 14:1;
24:3, 4).

God is your Partner as you prepare your
home for the new baby. One of the Old
Testament names of God is Jehovah-Jireh,
which means *"the Lord will provide."* "Your
Father knoweth what things ye have need of,
before ye ask him" (Matthew 6:8b). And he
knows what things will be needed by your
newborn child!

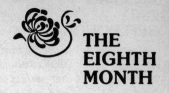

THE EIGHTH MONTH

Baby can weigh as much as 3 pounds, measuring 16 to 18 inches.

Lungs develop strength, and babies born this month have a good chance of survival. Skin is not so wrinkled, but still red. Protective covering *(vernix caseosa)* waterproofs the infant's skin.

You gave me skin and flesh and knit together bones and sinews. You gave me life and were so kind and loving to me, and I was preserved by your care.
Job 10:11, 12 (TLB)

REFINING
AND
REFLECTION

> *Cast thy burden upon the Lord, and he
> shall sustain thee . . . Let patience have
> her perfect work, that ye may be perfect
> and entire, wanting nothing.*
> Psalm 55:22; James 1:4

In these final weeks, your body is growing weary of the physical pressure of the child within.

You are exhausted from the effort it takes to get your cumbersome form out of bed, off of the sofa, or (cringe!) behind the wheel of your compact car. You're tired of not being able to sit close to the table, and sick of washing countless food stains off your protruding smock top.

You're tired of waddling instead of walking. Of getting up a dozen times each night to go to the bathroom. Of not being able to bend over and buckle your shoes. In fact, you'd be happy if you could even look down and *see* your shoes!

You've actually begun to wonder if the child within will *ever* become the child without!

Those who have never experienced the final months of a pregnancy laughingly misunderstand your fear that labor will never begin. Remember that you have an understanding heavenly Father. In Isaiah 66:9 (TLB), he reassures you, "Shall I bring to the point of birth and then not deliver? asks the Lord your God. No! Never!"

In these "pressing" days before delivery, as you faithfully go through your breathing exercises and relaxing drills, be faithful in exercising the spiritual quality of *patience*. "When the way is rough, your patience has a chance to grow. So let it grow. . . . For when your patience is finally in full bloom, then you will be ready for anything, strong in character, full and *complete*" (James 1:3, 4, TLB).

Complete. You're anxious for the arrival of your infant, but the work of the Holy Spirit is not yet completed!

You will never again have the joy of carrying *this* child within. Each succeeding pregnancy will be different. In the way he moves, the way he kicks, the way he lies within you, your baby is *already a unique individual.* Each day is an opportunity for the Holy Spirit to whisper something new to your heart about this special little person.

For years, scientists have tried to discover the answer to the question, "What causes labor to begin?" There are differing theories. Is it a hormone produced by the mother? A hormone from the glands of the baby? Or could it be the involuntary reaction of the abdominal muscles which have held the baby for as long as possible? Doctors are still unable to pinpoint when your labor will begin.

God alone knows your true due date. In his omniscience, he has specifically ordained, "A time to be born" (Ecclesiastes 3:2). In these last few days, he's adding a few "finishing touches" to the masterpiece you will soon hold in your arms! Don't be discouraged if baby overshoots his "estimated time of arrival." Your child may need a little more nutrition, a little more stamina. Like your spiritual growth, the physical growth of the child within must be, "Complete, wanting nothing."

No time in life need be wasted—not even your final weeks as a woman in waiting. How can this time be fulfilling? As the Lord brings to completion your baby's physical preparation for birth and your spiritual preparation for motherhood, you can look to the 37th Psalm for your "assignment." It would be wise to read this Psalm each morning (and perhaps memorize a portion of this passage); it is an excellent summary of all that has been covered in this study guide.

PSALM 37

I. v. 1—*"Fret not thyself . . ."*
    Review the Scriptures which will calm your fear and anxiety (chapter 4).

II. v. 3—*"Trust in the Lord, and do good."*
    Your "good work" is to complete the preparation of your home and marriage for the birth of your infant (chapter 7).

III. v. 4—*"Delight thyself also in the Lord."*
    "Seek ye first the kingdom of God . . ." (Matthew 6:33) by feeding your spirit through prayer and the Word (chapter 2).

IV. v. 5—*"Commit thy way unto the Lord."*
    Experience the sweetness of surrender to his will, knowing that his will flows out of his love. (chapter 1).

V. v. 7—*"Rest in the Lord, and wait patiently for him."*
Carry through on your self-discipline; stay physically rested. A storehouse of strength is needed for the labor which may begin at any time (chapter 5).

VI. v. 8—*"Cease from anger . . ."*
Instead of accepting emotional turmoil, claim emotional stability. Reign as a queen! (chapter 3).

VII. v. 34—*"Keep his way . . ."* or *"Keep traveling steadily along his pathway . . ."* (TLB).
Allow the Lord to continually increase your spiritual insight and wisdom (chapter 6).

Yes, dear sister, pregnancy at term is a time of pressure. (Literally!) But times of pressure can be our times of greatest inner growth. They are times of refining, and:

> *There is wonderful joy ahead, even though the going is rough for a while . . . trials are only to test your faith, to see whether or not it is strong and pure. It is being tested as fire tests gold and purifies it—and your faith is far more precious to God than mere gold.*
> 1 Peter 1:6, 7 (TLB)

> *He knoweth the way that I take: when he hath tried me [refined me], I shall come forth as gold.*
> Job 23:10

The gift of patience

1. The first phrase of Psalm 37:7 defines patience: *Be still or rest before the Lord*

2. When we are involved in pressure situations, we always long for a way out! Why does the Lord allow times of pressure? (See Hebrews 12:1.)

   so we can run w/ perseverance the race marked out before us

3. What will be the result of the trials, or tests, that come our way? There are several!

   a. 2 Corinthians 1:3, 4 *comfort*

   b. Isaiah 48:10 *refinement*

   c. Hebrews 12:11 *righteousness and peace*

The amazing truth

1. Besides the final weeks of pregnancy, are there any other pressing situations in your life with which you must deal at this time?

   _____

   _____

2. At times you may say, "I don't feel like I'm able to cope with this situation." Gain confidence as you study 1 Corinthians 10:13. (Paraphrase it here.)

   Your problem is not new. God is faithful; He won't put too much on you. He will provide a means of escape.

3. The amazing truth is that times of pressure can bring our greatest spiritual growth. Trace the four steps of growth, as listed in Romans 5:3-5.

a. _Suffering_   b. _perseverance_

c. _Character_   d. _hope_

In these last days of pregnancy
Which of the instructions of Psalm 37 is your greatest challenge?

fret not

Apply this area of need to the promises of 1 John 5:14 and Matthew 21:22.

FURTHER DEVOTIONAL READING

God initiates labor and knows your "due date." Job 28:24; Job 34:21; Psalm 22:9, 10; Psalm 71:6; Isaiah 40:27-31; Galatians 1:15

Contentment. Psalm 116:7; Isaiah 28:12; Jeremiah 6:16; Matthew 11:28; Luke 3:14; 1 Corinthians 7:20; ~~Ephesians 4:11~~; 1 Timothy 6:6; 1 Timothy 6:8; Hebrews 4:1-3

Patience. Ecclesiastes 7:8; Luke 21:19; Colossians 1:11; 1 Thessalonians 5:14; Hebrews 3:6; 6:15; James 1:3-8; James 1:~~14~~ 12

SUMMARY
Though you are still in a *waiting time,* no season of your life need be a *wasted time.*

The final days of your pregnancy can be a

time of special instruction from the Lord. You will love the story of an expecting couple, told in Judges 13:8, 9:

> *Then Manoah intreated the Lord, and said, O my Lord . . . teach us what we shall do unto the child that shall be born. And God hearkened to the voice of Manoah . . .*

Through his Holy Spirit, the Lord *does* speak to Christian mothers who seek him. Allow your response to parallel that of Mary:

> *But Mary kept all these things, and pondered them in her heart.*
>
> Luke 2:19

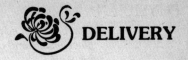

At term, the infant averages 4 to 8½ pounds.

The bones of the head remain soft and flexible to enable baby to pass through the birth canal. Child within "drops," head is in place, and baby is ready for birth. Labor may begin with contractions, mucus show, or with rupture of the "bag of waters."

When thou passeth through the waters,
I will be with thee . . .

Isaiah 43:2

MY GREAT
PHYSICIAN

*You both precede and follow me, and
place your hand of blessing on my head
[as I go].
I am holding you by your right hand—I,
the Lord your God—and I say to you,
Don't be afraid; I am here to help you.*
Psalm 139:5; Isaiah 41:13 (TLB)

There are two doctors who will assist in the
delivery of the child within. One is the
obstetrician you have chosen. The other is the
One whom Scripture names the "Great
Physician."

What a comfort to understand that besides
the hands of your doctor, there are gentle,
loving spiritual hands which will guide your
baby down the birth canal and into your
world! There are two verses from the Psalms
which beautifully portray the role of the Lord
in childbirth, especially if we look at these
verses in the original language, Hebrew.

In Psalm 22:9, 10, David said: "Thou art
he that took me out of the womb. . . . I was
cast upon thee from the womb: thou art my
God from my mother's belly." The word
"took" in the King James is translated from
the Hebrew word *gazah,* meaning "To pull,
or separate from; to cut." In this verse, God is
pictured as a skilled obstetrician assisting in
the birth, gently separating the baby from the
mother, and even cutting the umbilical cord.

In Psalm 71:6 we read, "By thee have I
been holden up from the womb; thou art he
that took me out of my mother . . ." The verb
"took" in this instance is actually the Hebrew
word *goach. Goach* means "working to bring
forth." *God will work with you throughout*

your labor and delivery. The beginning of the verse shows an especially touching scene, the Great Physician as he holds up the newborn for the inspection of the proud parents!

God is not only present when his daughters are in labor—he *understands* their labor and travail. Isaiah 42:14 tells us that he has *experienced* birth pangs as he endeavored to bring spiritual children into being.

As a child of God, you are not living under a "curse." During the Dark Ages, women were taught that God placed on Eve, and on all women, "the curse" of painful childbirth. This is *not* scriptural. In the King James version of Genesis 3:16 we read:

> *Unto the woman he said, I will greatly multiply thy sorrow and thy conception; in sorrow thou shalt bring forth children.*

Once again, let's look to the original language for a clearer understanding of this verse. The word translated as "sorrow" in the King James is the Greek word *esteb.* A much better translation of *esteb* would be "toil, labor, or hard work." The same word is used in Genesis 3:17 where God said to Adam, "In sorrow [*esteb*—with toil and labor] shalt thou eat of it [the ground] all the days of thy life." *Esteb is* translated as toil in other King James verses such as Genesis 5:29: "This same shall comfort us concerning our work and toil [*esteb*] of our hands . . ."

God literally told Eve, "In labor, with toil and work, you will bring forth children."

Instead of fearing this new experience, realize that the Word says what lies ahead of you is just plain work! That's what the word "labor" means, isn't it? It requires strength to carry out your breathing techniques, strength to refrain from bearing down too soon, and strength to push when the right time arrives!

Below is a general guide for the progression of labor, but the wise woman is mentally prepared for the *variations* labor can bring. Your labor may be relatively short or considerably long. The pangs may center in your abdomen or in your lower back. You may feel an almost uncontrollable urge to push—or you may not feel the urge at all. You may deliver naturally, as planned, or decide to use mild anesthesia. Though you have much in common with other women in waiting, your labor and delivery will be as unique as is the baby within you!

The miracle of birth.
1. THE FIRST STAGE OF LABOR:
    effacement and dilation—cervix is thinning and opening.
    Physical signs and changes: pink or red vaginal mucous "show"; possible back ache; possible rupture of membranes; regular uterine contractions that increase in strength, frequency, and duration.
    Emotions: excitement, anticipation, joy, energetic attitude.
    Wife's role: as need arises, begin to breathe with contractions.
    Remain calm as you are admitted and prepped.
    Use relaxation drills (entire body).
    Change position every half hour, empty bladder every half hour.
    Rest as much as possible between contractions.

*Rejoice! You're finally going to
receive the gift of your child within!

Husband's role: notify the doctor; at his
instructions, take your wife to the
hospital.

*Notify prayer partners and nearby
relatives.

Make sure your wife is comfortable.

Reassure her, give encouragement.

Remind her of the need to change
positions and empty bladder.

Place cool cloth on forehead, touch ice
to her lips (most hospitals won't
allow her to drink water).

Rub her back, give sacral pressure if
helpful.

Check with nurses on the progression
of labor after each exam.

*Pray for her, preferably out loud.

*Read to her from the Word.

A promise to claim: "The Lord will give
strength unto his people; the Lord will
bless his people with peace . . .
I will go in the strength of the Lord
God" (Psalm 29:11; 71:16).

2. TRANSITION: cervix dilating from 7 to
10 centimeters.

Physical signs and changes: (you may
feel some or all of these).
Increasingly strong contractions; possible back ache and soreness of abdomen; nausea; weariness; urge to
push; cheeks flushed (Malor flush);
chills.

Emotions: at 3-4 centimeters you
become more serious and may no
longer wish to talk; at 8-10 it is harder
to concentrate; you may feel ap-

prehension or fatigue, possible ir-
ritability.

Wife's role: breathing—use transition
drills.

Relaxation drills (of abdominal wall)—
rely on husband for help.

Rest whenever possible (a small dose
of medication, such as Demerol 50
mg. or Pethedine 50 mg., may be offered to help relaxation).

Continue to change positions and
empty bladder frequently.

*Claim God's peace, remember God's
presence!

Husband's role: time contractions,
deal with each one as it begins. Direct
breathing and relaxation drills (breathe
with her) and remind her to deep-
breathe between contractions.

Try backrub or sacral pressure.

Encourage her, assuring her she's doing well.

Act as a go-between for wife and staff;
protect her from confusion.

Get socks, blankets, if she is chilly.

Tell nurses when she feels the urge
to push, encourage her if she must
wait.

*Continue to intercede for her and
the baby.

A promise to claim: "I am holding you
by your right hand—I, the Lord your
God—and I say to you, Don't be
afraid; I am here to help you"
(Isaiah 41:13, TLB).

3. PUSHING: (beginning of second stage of
labor) mother cooperates with uterine
muscles to push baby down the birth
canal.

Physical signs and changes: tremendous urge to push, pressure of baby's head in vagina, feeling of warmth, possible body trembling.

Emotions: relief that now you can push, drowsy between contractions, excitement again builds.

Wife's role: assume pushing position— take two deep breaths, take one more, hold and bear down.

Cooperate with doctor; if you need to temporarily refrain from pushing, use panting drill.

Rest between contractions.

*Rely on the Lord for his strength.

Husband's role: hold up wife's shoulders if supports aren't available.

Remind her to relax between pushes.

Breathe with her, comfort her.

Tell her how well she's doing, cheer her on!

A promise to claim: "I can do all things through Christ which strengtheneth me" (Philippians 4:13).

4. DELIVERY OF THE CHILD!

Physical signs and changes: "pins and needles" sensation as vulva stretches; birth outlet becomes numbed (doctor may give a local anesthetic); discomfort becomes *less* than it was during transition and pushing.

Emotions: excitement, yet peace; laughing or crying with joy, awe and reverence.

Wife's and husband's roles: watch for baby's birth . . . enjoy it!

Your difficult work is over!

Encourage one another.

Listen for the first cry!

5. DELIVERY OF PLACENTA: (third stage of labor) placenta separates from uterine wall and moves down birth canal.

Physical signs and changes: one or more final contractions, stitches are taken to close episiotomy, you may feel hunger or thirst as soon as task is completed.

Emotions: tremendous joy, excited talking, probably wide-awake feeling with renewed energy.

Wife's role: Cuddle and enjoy your newborn (many hospitals suggest nursing immediately).
Thank your husband for his help.
Thank the doctors and nurses.
*Praise and thank the Lord!
Settle down for peaceful sleep.

Husband's role: congratulate your wife for a job well done.
Hold and enjoy your new baby.
*Praise and thank the Lord.
See your wife to the recovery room.
Make important *announcement* phone calls.
Get some well-earned rest.

> *And Jesus said, "Your weeping shall suddenly be turned to wonderful joy [when you see me again]. It will be the same joy as that of a woman in labor when her child is born — her anguish gives place to rapturous joy and all pain is forgotten."*

John 16:20, 21 (TLB)

"My help cometh from the Lord."

Psalm 121:2

1. What does God's Word promise regarding:
   a. His presence in time of need? (See Psalm 41:2; 145:18.) *He is near to all who call on Him*

   b. The amount of strength which is available to us? (See Deuteronomy 33:25.)

   _____

2. In Prepared Childbirth classes, women are encouraged to imagine a peaceful scene to facilitate relaxation in labor. Can you picture yourself in the beautiful illustration given in Isaiah 40:31: *soar on wings like eagles*

3. Study the divine help available in labor with regard to:
   a. your ability to concentrate (2 Timothy 1:7)

   self-discipline & power

   b. relaxation (Isaiah 28:12) *rest place of repose*

   c. speedy recovery (Jeremiah 30:17)

   _____

   _____

"I am the Lord that healeth thee."

Exodus 15:26

1. As a daughter of the Lord you are promised protection and safety. What do each of the following verses tell you about God's will for your physical well-being?

   a. Psalm 103:3, 4 _heals all my diseases_

   b. Isaiah 58:8 _healing will quickly appear_ (Chosen Fast)

   c. Zechariah 2:5 _____

2. Does the health promised to you apply to your baby as well?

   a. Deuteronomy 28:1-11 (esp. v. 4) _fruit of womb will be blessed_

   b. Psalm 107:15 _____

3. How does your Father respond to your prayers for your child? (See Isaiah 45:11.)

   He is the Creator

   _____

4. In your own words, describe the picture given in Joshua 33:12 of the way God will care for your infant.

   _____

"By a new and living way . . ."

Hebrews 10:20

1. As your contractions begin, remember that you are not bound to past experiences of mother, sister, or friends. What advice does Isaiah 43:18, 19 give to the woman in labor?

   Forget the past _He's doing a new thing._

2. Earlier in this chapter you read that you are *not* under a "curse" in childbirth.

What exciting truth do we find in 2 Corinthians 5:17-19? 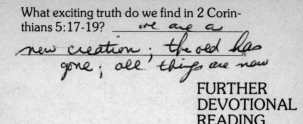 _we are a new creation; the old has gone; all things are new_

FURTHER DEVOTIONAL READING

Safety, strength, and protection.
Deuteronomy 33:12; Psalm 28:6-8;
Psalm 33:17-22; Psalm 34:7, 8;
Psalm 91:1-16; Proverbs 28:18; Isaiah 26:3;
Isaiah 30:15; Isaiah 40:31;
Isaiah 41:8-10, 13; John 10:10; John 16:21;
Philippians 4:19; 1 Timothy 2:15;
James 1:17

God's will—health. Psalm 42:11; Psalm 67:2;
Psalm 103:3; Psalm 107:20; Isaiah 53:5;
Malachi 4:2; Matthew 10:8; Luke 9:2; 10:9;
Acts 10:38; Acts 14:9; 1 Corinthians 12:9;
James 5:16; 1 Peter 2:24

SUMMARY

One of the titles the Word gives to the Lord Jesus parallels the experience which culminates your time as a woman in waiting—delivery. In Romans 11:26, as well as in many other beautiful portions of Scripture, we are told *"The Deliverer will come. . . "* (RSV).

Your Lord will be present as your Deliverer, as your Great Physician. He is with you not only to help you, but to rejoice with you!

> *The Lord thy God* in the midst of thee *is mighty; he will save, he will rejoice over*

99

thee with joy . . . he will joy over thee with singing.

Zephaniah 3:17

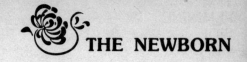 # THE NEWBORN

I have called thee by thy name;
thou art mine . . .

Isaiah 43:1b

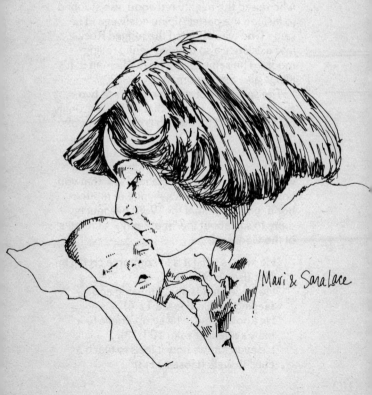

/Mari & Sara Lace

THE
FEMININE
SIDE
OF GOD

*Can a woman forget her suckling child,
that she should not have compassion on
the son of her womb? Yea, they may
forget, yet will I not forget thee!*

Isaiah 49:15

The same God who created the surging tides
and pounding surf of the ocean also designed
the woodlands through which sparkling
streams whisper his praise. The same God
who raised the mighty redwood also stooped
to fashion the pastel Alpine edelweiss. The
same God who shouted the rugged Rockies
into existence also molded gently rolling
moors. The same God who made man in his
image also made woman.

The spectrum of creation points to two
aspects of God's nature: that which is strongly
masculine, and that which is reminiscent of
femininity.

Before delivery, you studied Scriptures
which showed that the Lord identifies with a
woman's labor and birth pains. Now that you
have stepped into the challenge of motherhood, you'll find that the Word has much
more to say about the "mothering" attributes
of the Godhead.

* He knows what it is to comfort a crying infant (Isaiah 66:13).
* He understands about nursing and
  feeding a child (Hosea 11:4).
* He knows how to be sympathetic to a
  baby's needs (Psalm 103:13).
* He even knows how it feels to teach a
  child to walk (Hosea 11:3).

102

In Luke 13:34, we catch a glimpse of the heart of God when Jesus cried, "O Jerusalem, Jerusalem! . . . How often I have wanted to gather your children together even as a hen protects her brood under her wings . . ." (TLB).

By seeing the Scriptures' portrait of the tenderness of the Lord, you will grow to understand the *special divine presence* that is with a mother as she cares for her baby. The Bible has a beautifully descriptive word for God's tenderness. It is *lovingkindness.*

> *In lovingkindness, he is there to laugh with you as the nursing newborn tries to gobble you up!*

> *In lovingkindness, he is there to encourage you as you change diapers, wash diapers, then change them again. He says, "Let us not lose heart and grow weary and faint in acting nobly and doing right . . ."*
>   (See Galatians 6:9, Amplified)

> *In lovingkindness, he is there to stand guard with you as you take the "night watch" over a sick or restless baby.*
>   (See ~~Psalm 41:8, 63:6~~)

> *In lovingkindness, he is there to uphold you as you stumble to the nursery in the dim light of dawn for that early-morning feeding. "I can't even count how many times a day your thoughts turn towards me. And when I waken in the morning, you are still thinking of me!"*
>   Psalm 139:17b, 18 (TLB)

At times you may be troubled by ambivalence, a dividing of the emotions, during this postpartum period. There are favorable feelings toward the joyful tasks of cuddling and feeding baby—and there are negative feelings toward the overwhelming magnitude of your responsibility.

Sandy, one mother of a newborn, asked, "I'm adjusting well to the responsibility, but could there be something wrong with me? I don't feel the surge of love that I expected to feel for my baby." If this has troubled you, remember that <u>love is not only emotion—it is action. It includes a simple exercising of the will. Love is another step in the walk of faith. By faith, care for your newborn lovingly, and the surge of feeling will soon follow</u>. After all, the newborn may look like a little stranger, in spite of the fact that he was your child within for nine months! In a few short days, you will wholeheartedly say, "This is bone of my bone, and flesh of my flesh."

Both you and your husband will deal with some feelings of selfishness. Even when a child has been long planned and is dearly wanted, your style of living can't help but be interrupted. "Will we ever be able to do all those things we want to do?" you wonder. "What about the sacrifices of time and money we will be making for our children?"

Don't feel condemned by these thoughts—they simply mean that you see parenthood as reality and not just a fantasy. When troubled, remind yourself of the kingdom principle of *great gain through giving.*

In Matthew 10:39, Jesus told his disciples, "If you cling to your life you will lose it; but if you give it up for me, you will save it" (TLB). In the context of this chapter, he meant that some of those listening would lose their lives because of their faith and discover the greater treasure of eternal salvation. This verse can also apply to the quality of life you will find as you give yourself in service, for in Luke 6:38 (TLB) he said:

> *For if you give, you will get! Your gift will return to you in full and overflowing measure, pressed down, shaken together to make room for more, and running over. Whatever measure you use to give — large or small — will be used to measure what is given back to you.*

Mothering is the "givingest" task in the world . . . for the newborn baby cannot show a great deal of thanks. On the days when the job seems thankless, remember that as you give to your child it is as though you are giving unto the Lord. "If, as my representatives, you give even a cup of cold water to a little child, you will surely be rewarded" (Matthew 10:42, TLB). "When you did it [fed, helped, or clothed] to these my brothers you were doing it to me!" (Matthew 25:40).

God will add his blessing to the repetitive, routine tasks of motherhood. Jesus delighted in adding a miraculous touch to the everyday lives of everyday people . . . turning the commonplace into the extraordinary. He can turn water into wine! He can turn what would be daily drudgery into a school of joyful discipleship!

Besides physical care, what spiritual care can you provide for your newborn child?

First of all, it is certain that the name you chose for this baby was meaningful to you and your husband. According to our Jewish spiritual heritage, we know that the name chosen for a child had great significance. Israeli boys' names often included "el," which referred to the name of the Lord: Joel,

Daniel, Michael. Girls' names were often taken from beautiful objects in nature, such as Rachel (God's lamb).

Do you know the meaning of the name you have chosen? Excellent reference books are available today, some even including a verse from the Bible which relates to each name. As you intercede for your infant, you can pray that the characteristics of your baby's name become reality. It is not an illusion to believe that your child's name can even be God-given! We read of many instances in Scripture when God named infants before they were born. To your special baby, the Lord says *"I have called thee, by name, thou art mine!"*

Another important principle of spiritual care is the *dedication of your infant unto the Lord.* This can be done publicly (perhaps you have been present in church services when children were dedicated), or privately in your own home.

Basically, it is a time of verbally recognizing that this is God's child; a time of committing him to a loving heavenly Father; a time of asking for wisdom to raise him according to the plan of the Lord. In Israel, the *first place* a newborn was taken was to the house of the Lord for the ceremony of dedication. Like Hannah, at the dedication of Samuel, we can say, "For this child I prayed; and the Lord hath given me my petition which I asked of him. Therefore also I have lent him to the Lord; as long as he liveth he shall be lent to the Lord" (1 Samuel 1:27, 28).

Possessing the promises. The promises of God's Word are yours for the asking.

This month's Bible study is one of the most exciting you will ever experience, for it deals with the blessings that are available to your children. The mother of faith can claim health, happiness, wisdom, even prosperity for her little ones.

Most of all, you can claim for them the same abundant life which you have discovered in the Lord Jesus . . .

> I will pour out my spirit on your off-
>   spring,
> and my blessing on your descendants:
> and they will spring up among the grass
> like poplars by streams of water.
> This one will say, "I am the Lord's":
> and that one will call on the name of
>   Jacob;
> and another will write on his hand,
> Belonging to the Lord.
>   (See Isaiah 44:3b-5.)

FAITH BUILDERS

God's plan for my baby
The Word is a treasure chest of knowledge to show you how to raise the child God has given you. Study God's plan in regard to the following areas:

1. Discipline (1 Samuel 3:13; Proverbs 19:18; 29:17)

    Eli did not restrain his sons & was judged severely.
    Discipline produces hope & peace & delight

2. Training by example (Proverbs 22:6; 2 Timothy 1:5)

    Train a child in the way he should go, and when he is old he will not turn from it

3. Love and tenderness (Ephesians 6:4; Titus 2:4)

don't exasperate your kids but love them

4. Providing for (Ephesians 6:4)

training & instruction of the Lord

5. Spiritual teaching (Deuteronomy 6:7; Joshua 24:15)

Love the Lord Thy God

6. Forgiving them (Luke 15:20) *the prodigal returns*

God's hand on my baby
You'll rejoice as you discover the heritage your child receives by being born in a godly home. What may you believe God for in each of the following areas?

1. Material blessing (Psalm 37:25) *I've never seen the righteous forsaken or begging bread*

2. Joy (Psalm 149:2) _____

3. Truthfulness (Isaiah 63:8) _____

4. Favor with people (Proverbs 20:7; 1 Samuel 2:26)

_____

5. Emotional strength (Isaiah 54:13) *great will be your children's peace*

6. Salvation (Acts 2:39; 1 John 2:13) _____

"... *For the joy that a [child] is born* ..."
John 16:21.

1. Your baby is a living illustration of God's blessing on your life. You have just

studied the ways in which you are to give
to your child. Now consider what the
Word says your child will give to you!

Psalm 127, v. 3 _heritage & reward_

v. 4 _weaponry_

v. 5a _____

v. 5b _no shame w/ enemies_

Proverbs 17:6 _crown & pride_

Proverbs 31:28 _call her blessed_

2. A child can also have a spiritual impact
on his parents! What did the children's ac-
tions teach in each of these instances?

2 Chronicles 24:1 _was king of Israel_

1 Samuel 2:18 _ministering_

Matthew 21:15, 16 _praising God_

Isaiah 28:9 _____

3. In your journal, write a prayer request of
how you desire this child to bring you joy
in his lifetime. (An example of prayer for
a child's future: 1 Chronicles 29:19.)

give my child the whole-
hearted devotion to keep
God's commands, requirements
& decrees
to love God and be a servant of
the most High

FURTHER
DEVOTIONAL
READING

Dedication of children to the Lord.
Exodus 13:12; Numbers 3:13;

Deuteronomy 21:17; 1 Samuel 1:11;
Nehemiah 10:36; Luke 2:22

Examples of parental love and wisdom.
Genesis 18:19; Exodus 2:3; 1 Samuel 2:19;
1 Kings 2:1-4; 1 Kings 3:26; Psalm 78:3-8;
Matthew 15:22; Mark 5:23; Luke 15:20;
2 Timothy 1:5

Some days mothering is easy.
Some days it is not.
Always remember your Source.
As time goes by, recall these days of spiritual
preparation.
Reread your journal.
Review the Scriptures that became
"your own."

When you held the child within
you learned the reality of the phrase
"[He] shall gently lead those that are
with young."
In the years to come
the promise will be completed. . .
"He shall gather the lambs with his arms. . ."

(Isaiah 40:11)

BIBLIOGRAPHY

Birch, William G. *A Doctor Discusses Pregnancy.* Chicago: Budlong Press, 1976.

Clark, Ann, and Alfonso, Dyanne. *Childbearing: A Nursing Perspective.* Philadelphia: Davis Company, 1976.

Gillespie, Clark. *Your Pregnancy Month by Month.* New York: Harper & Row, 1977.

Hicks, Roy. *The Word of Faith.* Portland, Oregon: College Printing Service, 1969.

Liley, H.M.I. *Modern Motherhood.* New York: Random House, 1966.

Mitchell, Robert McNair. *Nine months to Go: A Medical History.* Philadelphia: J. B. Lippincott Company, 1960.

Nilsson, Lennart. *A Child Is Born.* Stockholm: Albert Bonniess Forlag, 1965.

Niswander, Kenneth R. *The Women and Their Pregnancies; A Statistical Compilation.* Philadelphia: Saunders, 1972.

Romney, Gray, Little, Merrill, Quilligan, and Strander. *Gynecology and Obstetrics: The Health Care of Women.* New York: McGraw Hill, 1975.

Strong, James. *The Exhaustive Concordance of the Bible.* New York: Abingdon Press, 1890.

Wessel, Helen. *The Joy of Natural Childbirth.* New York: Harper & Row, 1963.

Wight, Fred H. *Manners and Customs of Bible Lands.* Chicago: Moody Bible Institute, 1953.

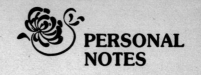

**PERSONAL
NOTES**